Points of Health

The Effectiveness and Safety of Acupuncture and Acupressure

Irwin Tyler

Ahl Kayn Publications
Spring Valley, NY

Points of Health

The Effectiveness and Safety of Acupuncture and Acupressure

ISBN 978-1-304-58021-4

First Printing - **2013**

Manufactured in the United States of America

TABLE OF CONTENTS

INTRODUCTION

Allopathic medicine (the kind of medicine your MD practices) has had a remarkable record of defeating disease and repairing a large variety of medical conditions. In the economically advanced countries average life expectancy has increased dramatically in the past 100 years (e.g. 25% in the United States). This is due in large part to advances in pre-natal and post-natal care. Antibiotics and advanced medical procedures also have been main drivers of this trend. But, just as one shoe size does not fit all, it doesn't make sense for there to be only one single system of healing that can successfully treat every known disease and condition. So, it isn't surprising that around the world we can find a number of very different, successful healing systems.

WELL, THEN, WHICH ONE SHOULD WE CHOOSE?

Within our human limitations, we can make informed and reasoned decisions about our own health care. We can look at the benefits of the many systems readily available to us and see which fits us best under different life circumstances and health conditions. For this reason, the booklet you are reading has been published.

LET'S LOOK AT THE HUMAN BODY

The body truly is a system, just as a car or airplane is a system. Damage one part and the entire system in one way or another becomes affected as well.

The body is not a series of functional parts. Remove a hand and it won't function on its own. Remove the thyroid gland and the body slows down and eventually will die. The medical literature presents countless examples of referred pain. There are reports of disabling pains in an arm or leg which ultimately trace back to a tooth infection. And many of us know of common sciatica, with its severe pain and/or numbness going down the leg to the knee or foot. But the problem is not in the foot or knee but is a pinched nerve at the spine. Clearly, what happens in one part of the body can affect other parts, sometimes in undetectable ways and sometimes in dramatic, serious ways.

Organs, themselves, are systems made up of countless individual cells. Impair a single cell in an organ and we take no notice of it. But impair enough cells and the function of the organ as a whole becomes impaired. We can't repair individual cells but we can enhance the body's ability to perform this repair work on each impaired cell. That is what healing is. The body is, in absolute fact, the only mechanism that truly heals (leaving for another setting the understanding of many people that God really is the ultimate healer). Western medicine, Eastern medicine, and various natural healing approaches are the body's healing assistants. All practitioners of the healing arts are assistants, supplying the tools that the body may use to bring about complete healing.

THE MODERN HEALER

According to Dr. David Williams, medical researcher, the amount of medical knowledge being published doubles every five years. How many doctors (allopathic healers) are able to spend the time to keep up with this massive wealth of new information?

Very simply, the modern healer has been forced to become a specialist because of the explosion of new healing information now becoming available. This creates the following situation: the modern healer becomes more expert about many fewer health concerns. In many cases this helps his patients greatly. Yet, sometimes it's more important to know about the total health concerns of his patients, about which he is less expert. And the healing solutions he may propose likely will not include safe, alternative healing solutions because he has little time outside of his specialty to research these other healing arts.

'So, what are my alternatives?'

WHAT ABOUT HOLISTIC MEDICAL PRACTICE?

Holistic medicine has a very special concern - preventing illness and maintaining health. Very simply, holistic medicine focuses on maintaining the health of the entire body. It views the body as parts that work together and that can not separately function in harmony. It views health as a balance of body systems - mental, emotional, and spiritual, as well as physical. While conventional medicine has a powerful arsenal of weapons to coax the ill body back to health, holistic medicine uses a wider range of therapies which reinforce the body's own defenses and restore balance.

Holistic medicine recognizes the human body's ability to resist assaults to the body, to balance internal organ systems, to repair damaged cells, and to heal injuries. This approach generally does not even recognize the existence of specific diseases. Practioners identify bodily imbalances that show a variety of symptoms. Their first instinct is to see what might be done to strengthen the body's natural resistance and healing agents so that they can act against the imbalances more effectively, thereby accomplishing a cure.

WHICH WAY SHOULD WE GO?

Should we abandon a medical system that is not perfect? Should we abandon a medical system that has proven its worth? Clearly, not. But there is an answer within the bounds of logic. And that answer is composed of two parts:

- That which is "provable" by the standards of science.
- That which tradition and history have demonstrated for hundreds, if not thousands of years.

The scientific community recently has funded studies to discover which other healing systems are effective and which are no more than traditions passed on for generations but which have shown little result as healing arts. Where has this finally led us?

The U.S. National Institutes of Health (NIH), for example, is funding studies to determine, scientifically, the effectiveness of:

Acupuncture as a treatment for depression, attention-deficit hyperactivity disorder, osteoarthritis, and postoperative dental pain

Hypnosis as a treatment for chronic low back pain and accelerated fracture healing

Ayurvedic herbals as a treatment for Parkinson's disease.

Biofeedback as a treatment for diabetes, low back pain, and face and mouth pain caused by jaw disorders

Electric currents to treat tumors

Imagery for asthma and breast cancer.

Magnetic fields for the treatment of certain cancers and neurological conditions and for alleviating pain

We now see in the medical arts a coming together of the world of science and the world of experience. In some cases we are seeing individuals combining several approaches in a single medical practice – for example, offices with MDs, Chiropractors, and Medical Massage Therapists. In other cases we are finding more acceptable the practice of single non-allopathic healing specialties – Acupuncturists or practitioners of Traditional Chinese Medicine, or Homeopaths.

Drawing on scientific studies, anecdotal stories, ancient traditions, and new information about how the body works, the modern patient integrates ALL knowledge in an effort to prevent and combat disease and to treat other conditions.

WHAT IS STANDARD MEDICAL PRACTICE?

While conventional medicine does talk about prevention of disease, it spends most of its time treating people after they become ill. It usually focuses on the patient's immediate symptoms, mainly the major symptoms. It considers that the main causes of illness are pathogens (bacteria or viruses) or biochemical imbalances. Scientific tests are heavily relied upon for diagnosis. Drugs, surgery, and radiation are among the key tools for dealing with the problems. Allopathy does recognize that many physical symptoms have mental components (for example, emotional stress might promote an ulcer or chronic headaches). However, its approach often is to suppress the symptoms, both physical and psychological, making the patient feel better while the body heals itself.

WHAT IS HOLISTIC MEDICAL PRACTICE?

Holistic medicine has a different focus - preventing illness and maintaining health. Very simply, holistic medicine focuses on maintaining, all at the same time, the health of the entire body, which consists of interrelated parts that can not separately function in harmony. It views health as a balance of body systems - mental, emotional, and spiritual, as well as physical. It looks at all symptoms, even those that have no obvious relationship to the patient's major complaints, looking for bodily imbalances. While conventional medicine has a powerful and growing arsenal of weapons to coax the ill body back to health, alternative medicine uses a wider range of therapies to bolster the body's own defenses and restore balance.

Holistic medicine recognizes the human body's ability to resist internal assault while it works at balancing internal cellular and organ systems and healing injuries. This approach generally does not even recognize the existence of specific diseases. The healer identifies bodily imbalances that exhibit a variety of symptoms. Their first instinct is to see what might be done to strengthen the body's natural resistance and healing agents so that they can act against the imbalances more capably, thus effecting a cure.

In this journal we are going to explore the rationale behind the better-known Acupuncture and its parent therapy, Acupressure, their strengths and weaknesses, and present some of their less understood successes (less understood from the allopathic standpoint).

UNDERSTANDING THE TERMS

Alternative Medicine

Alternative medicine is the current term applied to any healing art that is not part of conventional modern standard allopathic medicine. There are dozens of such healing philosophies, approaches, and therapies. Their diagnostic systems and understandings usually are different from that taught to their allopathic counterparts. Most of their understandings and methods are not taught in medical schools. Examples include: chiropractic, Ayurveda, and homeopathy. Practitioners of these healing arts usually practice only their own healing system, without reference to or consultation with a conventional allopathic healer. Their unique treatments are known as "alternative" medicine.

Complementary Medicine

When treatment or therapy includes some aspect of both allopathic and alternative treatments it is referred to as "complementary" medicine. In the West, some surgeons employ Acupuncture to reduce pain during surgery. In recent years specific lifestyle changes for the treatment of heart disease have been advocated by such practitioners as Dean Ornish. Qi Gong exercise is recommended by some allopathic healers as a therapy for hypertension. These are examples of the practitioners of complementary medicine.

Holistic Medicine

Many of the alternative practices pay attention to the mental, emotional, and spiritual aspects of health, in addition to the physical body. Practitioners believe that our bodies are remarkably resilient machines which are capable of healing themselves. Holistic alternative therapies like hypnosis and visualization have shown the ability to change physical conditions through purely mental intervention.

There are ancient healing practices of aboriginal tribes, the ancient Chinese and Japanese cultures, the American Indian and African Shaman healing Arts. All are based on the understanding that the body is a system and that all parts, especially the mental, emotional, and spiritual aspects of a person contribute both to the illness and its healing.

One can easily understand how the mind can play a major role in physical symptoms, since it is clear that hypochondriacs often experience real symptoms that have no established physical cause.

This role of the mind is just as meaningful in physical healing. Although not strictly Holistic Medicine, there is some recognition of the non-physical in modern medicine, where physicians sometimes will call on the "power" of the placebo effect to address the medical conditions of some of their patients. Hypnotism, too, has been used to some extent for addressing certain physical conditions.

Thus, we see that Western medicine does use the power of the mind, in some cases, to enhance the body's ability to heal itself. The reason that many forward-thinking Western medical practitioners will use such an "unorthodox" approach, with confidence, is because it works.

The name "holistic medicine" is this unification of the mind and the body. While modern allopathic medicine has become ever more divided into specialties, holistic practitioners treat the "whole person" as opposed to the individual organs of the body where symptoms occur. The importance of self care and preventing illness are stressed by holistic practitioners.

CAN WE TRUST THESE ALTERNATIVES?

These alternative health practices today are used by millions of people, and they have done so for thousands of years. Which is not to say that all alternative therapies are effective or safe. Which is not to say they work all the time, or for everyone. This is no different from our allopathic medical practices and therapies.

More and more, in this modern era, controlled studies of traditional healings reveal the effectiveness of alternative healing approaches. For many conditions, traditional healings are a useful assist to the allopathic practitioner. For many conditions for which allopathic practitioners have little to offer, traditional healings sometimes are the only effective treatment.

Gaining growing respect of the allopathic community are such traditional approaches as Acupuncture, Acupressure, TCM (Traditional Chinese Medicine), and Ayurvedic medicine (herbals), each of which has thousands of years of treatment history. In more modern times, Homeopathy and Chiropractic have shown great success for many conditions, both anecdotally from thousands of patients, and in recent controlled studies.

SECTION I - ACUPUNCTURE

THE ACUPUNCTURE MEDICAL UNDERSTANDING

Acupuncture is concerned with the whole person. It is the oldest, most commonly practiced medical procedure in the world and is used by one-third of the world as a primary healthcare system.

The report from a Consensus Development Conference on Acupuncture held at the National Institutes of Health (NIH) in 1997 stated that Acupuncture is being widely practiced by thousands of physicians, dentists, acupuncturists, and other practitioners for the relief or prevention of pain and for various other health conditions. Acupuncture finally has become widely accepted in the United States and has been endorsed by the World Health Organization (WHO) and the National Institutes of Health (NIH).

How Acupuncture Started

Acupuncture, derived from the earlier Acupressure therapy, originated in China, and its use dates back some 4,500 years. Chinese medicine, which incorporates Acupuncture into its many treatments, is considered to be the oldest and most widely used system of medicine in recorded history.

Acupuncture developed slowly and was well established when numerous medical authors around 475 to 221 BC contributed to The Nei Jing, also called The Yellow Emperor's Classic of Internal Medicine. It is the oldest medical book in China.

Acupuncture became fully accepted when, in the Tang Dynasty (618-907AD), medical academies were established and standard training methods and devices were developed for teaching the practice of Acupuncture.

Acupuncture in the Modern World

Beginning in the 17th Century and for the next 300 years there was a decrease in the practice of Acupuncture because of the increasing influence of Western ideas (allopathic medicine) in China.

Since the second World War, however, there has been a resurgence of Acupuncture in China, and a growing appreciation of its complementary role to Western medicine.

The year 1971 was a major turning point in the West. American commentator James Reston was visiting China when he was stricken with an acute appendicitis attack and required emergency surgery. Two days later, suffering from post operative abdominal pain, he was treated using Acupuncture and moxibustion at points near the knees and elbows. To his surprise he received considerable pain relief.

Following his recovery, he visited hospitals and communes. In many of them he found Acupuncture being used for a wide variety of conditions. Upon his return to the United States, his eye witness accounts were picked up by the public and the media. At one point he wrote, "I have seen the past, and it works".

As a result, many Westerners have begun to study the art of Acupuncture, and professional Acupuncture associations and schools have been established all over the world.

The Acupuncturist as Diagnostician

Allopathic diagnosticians look for groups of symptoms in order to identify and name a medical condition. Once named , treatments follow a standard protocol. Often the aim is to relieve symptoms as quickly as possible.

The acupuncturist takes a wider view. Acupuncture diagnostics is based on the view that natural laws describe the movement of energy in nature and the body. This life force, called Qi flows through the body in channels similar to rivers moving through earth. Health is promoted when the Qi in the body is full and moving properly. Illness can begin when the Qi is blocked in some manner.

There are two aspects to the Qi. Yin represents the cold, slow, or passive principle, while Yang represents the hot, excited, or active principle. Disease is due to an internal imbalance of Yin and Yang. This imbalance leads to blockage in the flow of Qi.

Acupuncture treats the underlying imbalances and promotes harmony within the body. When the body is in harmony, healing happens.

Blocked Qi can be unblocked by using Acupuncture at certain points on the body that connect with Qi pathways known as meridians.. One commonly cited source describes meridians as 14 main channels "connecting the body in a weblike interconnecting matrix" of at least 2,000 Acupuncture points.

What Modern Acupuncture Accomplishes

Acupuncture is said to be helpful for headaches, chronic fatigue, depression, allergies, back pain, digestive disorders, joint pain, sleeping problems, infertility, menstrual disorders and other symptoms. It is also said to be effective for severe chronic conditions where pinpointing the cause has been difficult to determine. Those who receive ongoing treatment for maintenance and the promotion of good health have reported that they:

- Tend to get sick less often and recover more quickly
- Have improved stamina and vitality

- Are better managers of their own health

- See reductions in long-term health care costs and tend to visit physicians less often

- Enjoy deepened, more harmonious relationships with others

Most of these claims are based on thousands of years of reported treatments in China. Western scientists are now studying the efficacy of Acupuncture and have begun to amass scientific confirmation of many of these claims, particularly those concerning pain (see reference citations below).

There is evidence that people's attitudes about Acupuncture can affect outcomes. In a 2007 study, researchers analyzed data from four clinical trials of Acupuncture for various types of chronic pain. Participants had been asked whether they expected Acupuncture to help their pain. In all four trials, those with positive expectations reported significantly greater pain relief.

How Acupuncture Works

Acupuncture still is the object of intensive study. The most commonly held theory in the West is the "Gate Control" theory. The "Gate Control" theory suggests that pain impulses are blocked from reaching the spinal cord or brain at various "gates" to these areas. A majority of Acupuncture points are located either near, or connected to neural structures. This suggests that Acupuncture stimulates the nervous system in a specific way that "shuts the gate" to the sensation of pain. Other Western theories suggest that Acupuncture stimulates the body to produce narcotic-like substances such as endorphins and opioids which, when released into the body, relieve pain.

The treatment process calls for special needles to be inserted just beneath the skin's surface at specific points on the affected "meridians".

The Acupuncture needles are slender - slightly thicker than a human hair - and are solid as opposed to hollow syringe needles. Typically used are high quality, stainless steel, pre-sterilized, disposable needles.

Non-needle Approaches

Moxabustion is the process whereby moxa - a dried herb, usually the species mugwort - is burned, either directly on the skin, or just above the skin, over specific Acupuncture points relative to a condition. When lit, moxa burns slowly and provides a penetrating heat that can enter the channels, or meridians to influence Qi and blood flow.

Cupping, the use of suction cups at Acupuncture points, is used in China today primarily to treat respiratory ailments such as asthma and bronchitis but is also used for arthritis, low back pain, depression, gastrointestinal problems and many types of pain in large soft tissue areas. Although often used as a therapy on its own, cupping often is used after an Acupuncture treatment to further stimulate the flow of blood and Qi to the area.

Gua Sha stimulates the underlying skin tissue without damaging the skin surface. Gua means to rub or friction. The term Sha describes congestion of blood at the surface of the body. A round-edged instrument is pressed on an oiled area in a firm scraping motion along the length of the muscle, or along the acupuncture meridians. This causes blood to evacuate the capillaries (petichiae). In minutes the petichiae fade into echymotic patches. The sha disappears totally in 2-3 days. The color and rate of fading are both diagnostic and prognostic indicators. Gua Sha removes metabolic waste that congests the surface tissues and muscles, and promotes the free flow of Qi and Blood. Gua Sha is used to treat fever, fatigue, poor circulation, respiratory distress, soft tissue injury or soreness, digestive disorders, general pain, and various diseases caused by functional disharmony of the internal organs, such as gynecological and urinary disorders, and any condition where palpation indicates there is sha.

The Evidence

A growing body of anecdotal evidence is available, many backed by studies in the West, showing effectiveness for:

- Pain. Back pain is the most commonly reported use, followed by joint pain, neck pain, and headache. There were promising findings by the American College of

Physicians in 2007 concerning back pain and some other conditions, such as osteoarthritis of the knee.

- Carpal tunnel syndrome — A 1997 NIH consensus statement on Acupuncture concluded that it was promising for this condition.
- Headache/migraine — A 2008 review of randomized trials on Acupuncture featured several well-designed trials whose findings indicate that Acupuncture reduces migraine symptoms and is as effective as headache medications.
- Menstrual cramps — Two literature reviews have suggested that Acupuncture may help with pain from menstrual cramps, but the research is limited.
- Myofascial pain — The evidence for Acupuncture and myofascial pain (in which pain occurs in sensitive areas, known as trigger points, in the muscles) is mixed. Some literature reviews have found the evidence promising, but another review indicated that "needling therapies" for myofascial trigger point pain were not more effective than placebo.

- Neck pain — Studies of Acupuncture for chronic neck pain have found that it provides better pain relief than some simulated treatments.
- Osteoarthritis/knee pain — Acupuncture appears to be effective for osteoarthritis, particularly in the area of knee pain. Recent literature reviews have found that Acupuncture provides pain relief and improves function for people with osteoarthritis of the knee.
- Postoperative dental pain — Although recent data on Acupuncture for postoperative dental pain are limited, literature reviews based on earlier evidence have identified Acupuncture as a promising treatment for dental pain—especially pain following tooth extraction. For example, a 1999 study of 39 dental surgery patients found that Acupuncture was superior to placebo (simulated Acupuncture) in preventing postoperative pain.
- Tennis elbow — Study results on the use of Acupuncture for tennis elbow (lateral epicondyle) pain have found the evidence promising, noting strong evidence that

Acupuncture provides short-term pain relief for lateral epicondyle pain.

- Pregnancy — Eric Manheimer of the University of Maryland School of Medicine's Center for Integrative Medicine and colleagues found that Acupuncture given as a complement to in-vitro fertilization increased the odds of achieving pregnancy.
- Nausea/vomiting — These conditions often accompany other treatments. Acupuncture has been helpful in many cases in reducing or relieving completely the antiemesis resulting from these treatments.
- Hypertension — Acupuncture has been effective in many cases of hypertension, backed by early study results. These studies showed Acupuncture influencing blood pressure regulating hormones, reducing renin, angiotensin II, and aldosterone levels, and increasing serum nitric oxide (NO).

The World Health Organization recognizes Acupuncture as an effective treatment for:

- **Digestive disorders:** gastritis and hyperacidity, spastic colon, constipation, diarrhea.

- **Respiratory disorders:** sinusitis, sore throat, bronchitis, asthma, recurrent chest infections.
- **Neurological and muscular disorders:** headaches, facial tics, neck pain, rib neuritis, frozen shoulder, tennis elbow, various forms of tendinitis, low back pain, sciatica, osteoarthritis.
- **Urinary, menstrual, and reproductive problems.**

Numerous published reports by the UK Acupuncture Research Resource Centre reveals effective treatments for, stroke, menopause, addiction and substance abuse, anxiety and depression – to cite just a few conditions amenable to Acupuncture therapy.

Selected Study Citations

National Institutes of Health Consensus Panel. Acupuncture: *NIH Consensus Development Conference Statement, Nov. 3–5, 1997.* 15(5):1–34.

Madsen MV, Gøtzsche PC, Hróbjartsson A. *Acupuncture treatment for pain: systematic review of randomized clinical trials with*

Acupuncture, placebo Acupuncture, and no Acupuncture groups. BMJ. 2009;338:a3115.

Zhang Y, Liu YX, Pan KY. The comparative study on the effects of Acupuncture, moxibustion and the combination on the renin-angiotensin-aldosterone system and cardionatrin levels. *Journal of Hubei College of Traditional Chinese Medicine.* 2001;3(2):20-21.

Yang, et al. *Ovulation induction for hormonal infertility.* Acupuncture Research Resource Centre, British Acupuncture Council. 2005

Harris RE, Tian X, Williams DA, et al. *Treatment of fibromyalgia with formula Acupuncture: investigation of needle placement, needle stimulation, and treatment frequency.* Journal of Alternative and Complementary Medicine. 2005;11(4):663–671.

Furlan AD, van Tulder M, Cherkin D, et al. *Acupuncture and dry-needling for low back pain: an updated systematic review within the framework of the Cochrane collaboration.* Spine. 2005;30(8):944–963.

Trinh KV, Graham N, Gross AR, et al. Cervical Overview Group. *Acupuncture for neck disorders.* Cochrane Database Systematic Reviews. 2006;3:CD004870.

Kwon YD, Pittler MH, Ernst E. *Acupuncture for peripheral joint osteoarthritis: a systematic review and meta-analysis.* Rheumatology (Oxford). 2006;45(11):1331–1337.

Goldman RH, Stason WB, Park SK, et al. *Acupuncture for treatment of persistent arm pain due to repetitive use: a randomized controlled clinical trial.* The Clinical Journal of Pain. 2008;24(3):211–218.

Lee A, Done ML. *The use of nonpharmacologic techniques to prevent postoperative nausea and vomiting: a meta-analysis.* Anesth Analg 1999;88(6):1362-9.

Orman D, Meargetis D: *Effectiveness of Acupuncture and Chinese Phytomedicinals in the treatment of HIV and AIDS.* J NaturopathicMed 1992; 3(1): 80-81

WHY TRY ACUPUNCTURE

Ann Fonfa, President of the Annie Appleseed Project (providing information, education, advocacy, and awareness about complementary or alternative medicine (CAM) and natural therapies since 1999) has been spreading the following message to medical societies, symposiums, and conferences worldwide:

> "Even if the workings of a natural substance or technique cannot be fully explained, that does not diminish the reality of its effect."

Chinese and other Asian experience with Acupuncture has demonstrated for millions of people its usefulness as a healing art. Whether Acupuncture operates on "gates", or enhances the placebo effect, or excites narcotic-like production, modern studies are verifying the 3,000 year old Chinese traditions showing the value of Acupuncture as a medical treatment.

To sum up, Acupuncture care is a cost-effective alternative to the management of many challenging health conditions. It is increasingly accepted by the public and there is a growing body of evidence that patients prefer Acupuncture over other forms of care for those conditions proven, to this date, to be responsive to this treatment protocol.

There is every reason to believe, based on recent Western studies, that Acupuncture will be "proven" to be more useful for many more medical conditions than currently understood in the West.

SECTION II – ACUPRESSURE

THE ACUPRESSURE MEDICAL UNDERSTANDING

Acupressure is concerned with the whole person. It uses the fingers, and sometimes the feet, to press key points on the surface of the skin to stimulate the body's natural self-curative abilities. In its own terminology, it channels the body's healing energy / life force.

The Chinese call this healing energy Qi (Chi). In Japan, the life force is termed Ki, and channeling healing energy is called Reiki. Yoga practices refer to the body's life force as prana or pranic energy. These terms all relate to the same universal healing energy.

In some traditional Asian medical philosophies, health is considered to be a state of balance in the body, maintained by the flow of life energy along specific meridians. The philosophy that disease is caused by imbalance has led to treatments directed at establishing balance through points along these meridians. Disease is believed to occur when there is blockage in the flow of energy or when energy flow is deficient or in excess.

Acupressure points (also known as potent points) are sensitive locations on the skin. Stimulating these points with pressure, needles, or heat triggers the release of endorphins, the neurochemicals that relieve pain. As a result, pain is blocked and the flow of blood and oxygen to the affected area is increased. As an Acupressure point is pressed, muscle tension is thought to yield to the pressure, enabling muscle fibers to elongate and relax. This also allows the release of toxins from the affected area. Acupressure aims to restore this normal flow of life energy by means of finger pressure, palm pressure, stretching, massage and other techniques. There are said to be 12 primary channels and eight additional pathways that circulate life energy through the body, maintaining the balance of yin and yang. 365 pressure points are identified in most of the literature.

The stimulation of one Acupressure point can send a healing message to other parts of the body through the interconnected meridiens. In this way, each Acupressure point can address more than one complaint or symptom.

Acupressure's Beginnings

Acupressure originated in China, and its use dates back about 5,000 years, to emperor Huang Ti's reign. Chinese medicine, which incorporates Acupressure into its many treatments, is thus considered to be the oldest and most widely used system of medicine in recorded history. When Acupuncture was discovered to work similarly using needles, it became more popular. Although known around the world, today it is most often practiced in China, India, Japan, and Korea.

It was not until the 17th century that the western world became aware of Chinese medicine and Acupressure. The recent history of Acupressure reveals that the 1970s World Health Organization, after a series of research studies, declared Acupressure medicine highly effective in treating 40 major diseases

Acupressure in the Modern World

Acupressure is now increasingly recognized for curing pain and illness across the world. It is the 3rd most popular method for pain and illness relief in the world. Acupressure is widely practiced both professionally and informally throughout Asia for relaxation, for the promotion of wellness and for the treatment of disease. The major advantage of Acupressure in practice is that self-treatment is possible with Acupressure but not with Acupuncture.

A number of benefits of Acupressure have been noted:

- Can relieve pain in many cases no matter what the cause.
- Promotes overall well-being
- An adjunct to psychotherapy in removing tensions that interfere with that therapy
- Can speed the healing of fractures
- Makes Chiropractic spinal adjustments easier and more effective
- As a beauty treatment improving skin tone and lessening the appearance of facial wrinkles

- Is non-invasive and there are no negative side-effects.
- Is safe, easy to learn and do on oneself at home.

Traditional Chinese medicine (TCM) discovered that excesses of various activities weaken the immune system by overstressing certain Acupressure meridian pathways. Regular Acupressure point therapy and relaxation techniques can counteract stresses, prevent fatigue, and boost the immune system.

Acupressure is often combined with Reflexology, the stimulation of nerve endings in the hands and feet. This combination often is more effective than each alone.

Clearly, Acupressure is a system with many facets to it, being useful alone as well as an adjunct to other treatments.

The year 1971 was a major turning point in the West. American commentator James Reston was visiting China when he was stricken with an acute appendicitis attack and required emergency surgery. Two days later, suffering from post operative abdominal pain, he was treated using Acupuncture and moxibustion at points near the knees and elbows. To his surprise he received considerable pain relief.

Following his recovery, he visited hospitals and communes. In many of them he found Acupuncture being used for a wide variety of conditions. Upon his return to the United States, his eye witness accounts were picked up by the public and the media. At one point he wrote, "I have seen the past, and it works".

Following on the heels of Acupuncture, its predecessor therapy, Acupressure, was "discovered" in the West.

The Acupressure in Diagnosis

Allopathic diagnosticians look for groups of symptoms in order to identify and name a medical condition. Once named, treatments follow a standard protocol. Often the aim is to relieve symptoms as quickly as possible.

The Acupressure practitioner takes a wider view. Local symptoms are considered as a materialization of the condition of the body as a whole. Acupressure diagnostics is based on the view that natural laws describe the movement of energy in nature and the body. This life force, called Qi flows through the body in channels similar to rivers moving through earth. Health is promoted when the Qi in the body is full and moving properly. Illness can begin when the Qi is blocked in some manner.

The West recognizes two pulses, usually in the wrist and ankle, and sometimes another in the neck. Acupressure recognizes 9 different pulses. These are indicators of the state of Qi in different parts of the body and its organs.

There are two aspects to the Qi. Yin represents the cold, slow, or passive principle, while Yang represents the hot, excited, or active principle. Disease is due to an internal imbalance of Yin and Yang. This imbalance leads to blockage in the flow of Qi.

Acupressure treats the underlying imbalances and promotes harmony within the body. When the body is in harmony, healing happens.

Blocked Qi can be unblocked by using Acupressure at certain points on the body that connect with Qi pathways known as meridians. One commonly cited source describes meridians as 14 main channels "connecting the body in a weblike interconnecting matrix" of at least 2,000 Acupressure/Acupuncture points. Just as a dam may cause flooding upstream, blocked Qi may cause symptoms distant from the blockage point.

What Modern Acupressure Accomplishes

Acupressure is said to be helpful for backaches, arthritis, muscle aches, and anxiety and tension due to stress. Ulcer pain, menstrual cramps, lower back aches, constipation, and indigestion also respond well to Acupressure. Insomnia and headaches caused by these conditions are also thereby relieved.

Those who receive ongoing treatment for maintenance and the promotion of good health have reported that they:

- Tend to get sick less often and recover more quickly
- Have improved stamina and vitality
- Are better managers of their own health
- See reductions in long-term health care costs and tend to visit physicians less often

- Enjoy deepened, more harmonious relationships with others

Most of these claims are based on thousands of years of reported treatments in China. Western scientists are now studying the efficacy of Acupressure and have begun to amass scientific confirmation of many of these claims, particularly those concerning pain (see reference citations below).

How Acupressure Works

In traditional Chinese medicine, the meridians are channels in the body believed to conduct Qi, or elemental forces.

Acupressure points have a high electrical conductivity at the surface of the skin, allowing for effective channeling of this healing energy. In common with Acupuncture, Acupressure uses the use the same pressure points and meridians as Acupuncture, but Acupressure uses gentle to firm finger pressure. Different massage systems vary in their rhythms and pressures for stimulating the Acupressure points. Some use only the fingers, others also use the hands, arms, legs and even feet.

When these Acupressure points are stimulated, they release muscular tension, promote circulation of blood, and enhance the body's life force energy to aid healing.

Acupressure still is the object of intensive study. The most commonly held theory in the West is the "Gate Control" theory. The "Gate Control" theory suggests that pain impulses are blocked from reaching the spinal cord or brain at various "gates" to these areas. A majority of Acupressure points are located either near, or connected to neural structures. This suggests that Acupressure stimulates the nervous system in a specific way that "shuts the gate" to the sensation of pain. Other Western theories suggest that Acupressure stimulates the body to produce narcotic-like substances such as endorphins and opioids which, when released into the body, relieve pain.

Some symptoms are relieved almost immediately, while others may take some time to see a positive change.

Acupressure Approaches

Acupressure is a non-needle procedure utilizing finger pressure over the specific points on the affected "meridians". These are the same points utilized in needle Acupuncture. Typical techniques are: firm pressure, kneading, brisk rubbing, and tapping.

Shiatsu is the traditional Japanese form of Acupressure. Its literal translation is finger (shi) pressure (atsu). Shiatsu emphasizes finger pressure not only at acupoints but also along the body's meridians. Shiatsu can also incorporate palm pressure, stretching, massage and other manual techniques. This form of Acupressure can be intense, with deep pressure applied to each point for three to five seconds. In another form, Jin Shin Acupressure, at least two points are gently held for a minute or more.

Tuina (Chinese for "pushing and pulling") is similar to shiatsu, but it places more emphasis on soft-tissue manipulation and structural realignment. Tuina is reported as being the most common form of Asian bodywork practiced in Chinese-American communities.

The Evidence

A growing body of evidence is available, many backed by studies in the West, showing effectiveness for a variety of conditions:

J Perioper Pract. 2008 Dec;18(12):543-51. *Acupressure and acupuncture in preventing and managing postoperative nausea and vomiting in adults.*
Abraham J.
Faculty of Health and Life Sciences Coventry University, Coventry, CV1 5FB.

Acupressure Relieves Low Back Pain
ScienceDaily (Feb. 17, 2006) — Acupressure (applying pressure with the thumbs or fingertips to the same points on the body stimulated in acupuncture) seems to be more effective in reducing low back pain than physical therapy, finds a study published online by the British Medical Journal.

Acupressure conferred an 89% reduction in disability compared with physical therapy, after adjusting for pre-treatment disability. This improvement lasted for six months.

Acupressure Calms Children Before Surgery
ScienceDaily (Oct. 1, 2008) — An acupressure treatment applied to children undergoing anesthesia noticeably lowers their anxiety levels and makes the stress of surgery more calming for them and their families, UC Irvine anesthesiologists have learned.

J Pain Symptom Manage. 2008 Nov;36(5):529-44. Epub 2008 Apr 28. *Review of acupressure studies for chemotherapy-induced nausea and vomiting control.*

Lee J, Dodd M, Dibble S, Abrams D.
School of Nursing, University of California, San Francisco, California 94143, USA. jiyeon.lee@nursing.ucsf.ed
Suggestive effects of acupressure, cost-effectiveness, and the noninvasiveness of the interventions encourage researchers to further investigate the efficacy of this modality.

A nationwide survey in England found that shiatsu practitioners most commonly treat musculoskeletal and psychological conditions, including neck, shoulder and lower back problems; arthritis; depression; and anxiety.

Study Shows Acupressure Effective In Helping To Treat Traumatic Brain Injury
Article Date: 02 Mar 2011 - 0:00 PDT
A new University of Colorado Boulder study indicates an ancient form of complementary medicine may be effective in helping to treat people with mild traumatic brain injury, a finding that may have implications for some U.S. war veterans returning home.

In addition to recent studies, Acupressure practitioners are usually happy to show new patients testimonials from hundreds of their patients extending over many years. Science often dismisses this kind of anecdotal "evidence" yet these positive testimonials continue to accumulate over time.

Acupressure has been recognized by the World Health Organization (WHO) as a science that that works by activating neurons in the nervous system to stimulate the endocrine glands and activate the defective organ.

WHY TRY ACUPRESSURE

It's worth being reminded of the words of Ann Fonfa, President of the Annie Appleseed Project (providing information, education, advocacy, and awareness about complementary or alternative medicine (CAM) and natural therapies since 1999) has been spreading the following message to medical societies, symposiums, and conferences worldwide:

> "Even if the workings of a natural substance or technique cannot be fully explained, that does not diminish the reality of its effect."

Chinese and other Asian experience with Acupressure has demonstrated for millions of people its usefulness as a healing art. Whether Acupressure operates on "gates", or enhances the placebo effect, or excites narcotic-like production, modern studies are verifying the 5,000 year old Chinese traditions showing the value of Acupressure as a medical treatment.

To sum up, Acupressure care is a cost-effective alternative to the management of many challenging health conditions. It is increasingly accepted by the public in the West.

There is every reason to believe, based on recent Western studies, that Acupressure, like the better-known Acupuncture, will be "proven" to be more useful for many more medical conditions than currently understood in the West.

www.ingramcontent.com/pod-product-compliance
Lightning Source LLC
Chambersburg PA
CBHW050345290526
45785CB00006B/2635